JASON ROGERS

Living With Type 2 Diabetes

A guide for reducing blood sugar and living a healthy life

This book was professionally typeset on Reedsy.
Find out more at reedsy.com

Contents

1

Introduction

Welcome to *Living With Type 2 Diabetes*! My name is Jason Rogers. I'm very excited to share all of the information I've learned in my day to day struggle with Type 2 diabetes. I was diagnosed with Type 2 diabetes approximately 2 years ago. When I was diagnosed I was shocked! I ate fairly healthy. I didn't drink soda at all. I ate very little candy. How could this possibly happen? Looking back, there were several factors working against me. It started when I became completely stressed out about my car wash business. More elaborate car washes popped up in town and business got slow. Real slow. I ate to deal with the stress and gained weight until I was 280 lbs. I became tired all the time, sleeping almost as soon as I sat down to relax. My vision became blurry every now and again, lasting a few minutes each time it happened. I was always thirsty. Every night I would wake up at least 3 times, having to go to the bathroom. It wasn't until my sister jokingly asked if she could take my blood sugar levels that I realized I was in trouble. What my sister saw when the reading popped up made her eyes open wide! She said "256! You need to go see a doctor!" I didn't really know what this number meant until my doctor stated the normal range is anywhere from 70-100 mg/dL. He told me it was high but, not to worry, with medication and some lifestyle changes I would be able to get it under control. This began my journey of educating myself on all topics related to Type 2 diabetes.

A diagnosis of Type 2 diabetes presents a major hurdle for any-one—one that demands our attention and understanding. If you're reading this, it's likely that you've recently been diagnosed or are supporting someone who has. Don't worry, within this short book, I'll present a framework to navigate the twists and turns of living with Type 2 diabetes.

Living with Type 2 Diabetes is not your typical medical book; I am not a medical professional. This book is just a short, condensed collection of everything I've learned about Type 2 diabetes up to this point. I'm proud to share all my knowledge and hope you use this book as your compass to understanding and thriving with this condition. Here, I've included the essential knowledge you need into a concise guide, free from unnecessary jargon and fluff. I'm here to educate you with the wisdom to make informed choices and take control of your health journey.

In this book, we'll clear up most questions surrounding Type 2 diabetes, providing you with strategies to manage and even conquer it. From dietary shifts that can transform your daily life to the profound impact of exercise and sleep on your well-being, we'll get into the lifestyle changes that can help you reclaim control over your blood sugar levels.

We'll discuss the ever-elusive goal of weight management and stress reduction, recognizing the profound effects these factors can have on your health. You'll gain insight into the array of medications and supplements at your disposal, equipping you with knowledge to make informed decisions about your treatment.

Perhaps most crucially, we'll take a look at the complexity of blood glucose management—studying the science, exploring the tools, and offering practical advice to help you maintain steady, healthy levels throughout the day. We will go into detail about testing procedures, timing of testing, and the different methods of testing available to us.

By the time you reach the final pages of this book, you won't merely be informed; you'll be armed with a powerful toolkit to enhance your quality of life and take charge of your health narrative. So, let's embark on this journey together. Welcome to a life of thriving with Type 2 diabetes.

2

What Is Type 2 Diabetes?

I n this chapter, we'll examine Type 2 diabetes further, breaking down complex concepts into easily digestible insights that will give you a fighting chance to manage this condition effectively. In the United States alone, it's estimated that approximately 34.2 million people have diabetes, and the majority of these cases are Type 2 diabetes. Globally, the prevalence of diabetes has been steadily increasing, with over 463 million adults living with diabetes in 2019, according to the World Health Organization..

Definition

Type 2 diabetes is a metabolic disorder that significantly influences how your body handles glucose, the essential fuel for your cells. Unlike Type 1 diabetes, which stems from the body's inability to produce insulin altogether, Type 2 diabetes hinges on a different problem – insulin resistance. This means your body still produces insulin, but it struggles to use it efficiently. Consequently, your blood sugar levels can rise to unhealthy heights.

Causes

The causes of Type 2 diabetes often intertwine with lifestyle choices. Carrying excess weight, particularly around the abdominal area, and leading a sedentary life are significant risk factors. According to the Centers for Disease Control and Prevention (CDC), about 34.5% of American adults are obese, which is a significant risk factor for developing Type 2 diabetes. Your dietary choices also play an important role; a diet high in sugars and unhealthy fats can substantially increase your vulnerability. Having a family history of Type 2 diabetes can increase your risk as well. While genetics can lay the groundwork, your daily decisions hold the power to tip the scales either way. This means that, fortunately, you can lower your risk through conscious lifestyle adjustments.

Recognizing the Symptoms of High Blood Sugar

Think of your body as a finely-tuned instrument. When your blood sugar levels become too high, it's like an off-key note in an otherwise harmonious melody. Detecting the symptoms of high blood sugar early is like recognizing that off-key note. Keep an eye out for common signs, such as an unquenchable thirst, frequent trips to the bathroom, persistent fatigue, and occasionally, blurred vision. I suffered from all of the symptoms at some point. These early warning signals provide essential insights into your body's condition, enabling you to take swift corrective action. Ignoring these signals may lead to a more serious condition of being insulin dependent.

High/Low Glucose Numbers

Your blood sugar numbers act as a gauge, telling you how your body is performing. When your glucose numbers soar, it indicates hyper-glycemia, while low numbers signal hypoglycemia. Understanding these ranges and what they mean is like learning a new language – it opens up a direct line of communication with your body. Ideally, blood glucose should be in the range of 70-100 mg/dL. Currently, my numbers lie in the 90-120 mg/dL range. We need to use these numbers to decide how we should respond if we stray from the optimal path.

After reading this short chapter you should have a better understanding of what Type 2 diabetes is, what leads to its development, and how to recognize the signs of fluctuating blood sugar levels. Armed with this foundational knowledge, you'll be well-prepared to tackle the lifestyle changes and strategies outlined in the upcoming chapters. Your journey to thriving with Type 2 diabetes begins with a solid grasp of its fundamentals.

3

Changing Your Diet

In this chapter, we'll discuss practical dietary changes that can be transformative in managing Type 2 diabetes. Let's break it down with a few examples and facts.

Decreasing Carbohydrate Consumption

Carbohydrates are a primary source of glucose in your diet. For instance, a single cup of cooked pasta contains about 25 grams of carbohydrates. Instead of cutting carbs entirely, you'll learn to distinguish between simple and complex ones. Simple carbs like a 12-ounce can of soda can deliver a staggering 39 grams of sugar, causing rapid blood sugar spikes. Complex carbs, like a cup of cooked quinoa with 39 grams of carbohydrates, release glucose gradually. You'll discover how to calculate your daily carbohydrate needs based on factors like your activity level and manage your intake by focusing on nutrient-dense options, such as swapping white rice for quinoa and replacing sugary snacks with whole fruits.

Avoiding Simple Sugars

Sugar can be stealthy in your diet. For instance, a seemingly healthy yogurt cup can pack up to 15 grams of added sugar. By reading labels closely, you can spot hidden sugars in condiments like ketchup (a single tablespoon contains about 4 grams of sugar) or granola bars (some have up to 20 grams of sugar per serving). Instead of sweetening your coffee with sugar, you can opt for cinnamon, which has zero grams of sugar and adds flavor without the blood sugar spike. Recognizing that the sugar in fruit is natural and accompanied by fiber helps you make informed choices.

Embracing Good Fats

Good fats can be a game-changer in your diet. For example, avocados are a rich source of healthy fats; a typical avocado contains around 21 grams of monounsaturated fats. You can incorporate good fats by sauteing vegetables in olive oil, a tablespoon of which has 14 grams of monounsaturated fats. Snacking on a handful of almonds, which are packed with healthy fats and only 1 gram of saturated fat per ounce, can be a satisfying choice. Practical cooking tips, such as using unsaturated oils (olive oil, canola oil) can be a game-changer in your diet. For example, avocados are a rich source of healthy fats; a typical avocado contains around 21 grams of monounsaturated fats. You can incorporate good fats by sauteing vegetables in olive oil, a tablespoon of which has 14 grams of monounsaturated fats. Snacking on a handful of almonds, which are packed with healthy fats and only 1 gram of saturated fat per ounce is a great choice. Using these good-fat options for dressings and dips, will help you maximize the benefits of these fats.

Diets Suited for Type 2 Diabetes

Specific diets can align with Type 2 diabetes management. For example, the Mediterranean Diet emphasizes whole grains, vegetables, and lean proteins. A typical Mediterranean meal might include grilled chicken breast, a generous salad with olive oil dressing, and a side of quinoa. The Low-Carb High-Fat (LCHF) diet restricts carbohydrate intake while encouraging fats and proteins. A day on this diet might involve a breakfast of scrambled eggs with avocado and spinach, followed by a lunch of grilled salmon with asparagus and a side of cauliflower mash. These practical examples illustrate how to structure meals in line with these diets, offering satisfying and diabetes-friendly options.

Now you should have a better grasp of how to make specific dietary changes for managing Type 2 diabetes. With these examples and facts, you'll be equipped to decrease carbohydrate consumption, avoid hidden sugars, embrace good fats, and explore diets tailored to Type 2 diabetes. Knowing this, you can confidently make choices that help regulate your blood sugar levels while enjoying delicious and healthful meals.

4

Sleep and Exercise

This chapter sheds light on the relationship between sleep and exercise in the context of Type 2 diabetes management. Let's explore the effects of both and offer practical insights for your well-being.

Effects of exercise and sleep on Type 2 diabetes.

Exercise and sleep exert direct and measurable impacts on Type 2 diabetes. For instance, regular physical activity enhances insulin sensitivity, allowing your body to use glucose more efficiently. This leads to improved blood sugar control. Adequate sleep, on the other hand, regulates hormones affecting your appetite and blood sugar levels.

How much exercise is needed?

The American Heart Association recommends a minimum of 150 minutes of moderate-intensity exercise weekly. To put this into perspective, brisk walking for just 30 minutes a day, five days a week, meets this guideline. Alternatively, 75 minutes of vigorous-intensity exercise, like running or cycling, can yield similar benefits. Incorporating strength training exercises, such as resistance bands or body weight workouts, twice a week further enhances muscle health and blood sugar regulation.

What type of exercise is best?

The choice of exercise should align with your preferences and goals. Cardiovascular activities, like swimming or biking, promote overall health and contribute to better blood sugar management. Flexibility and balance exercises, such as yoga or tai chi, reduce the risk of injury. Resistance training, involving exercises like squats and push-ups, not only helps maintain muscle mass but also supports blood sugar control.

How much sleep is needed?

Adults typically require 7-9 hours of sleep per night for optimal health. This duration allows your body to complete essential sleep cycles. These cycles are crucial for various bodily functions, including hormone regulation, which affects blood sugar.

Improving sleep

Enhancing sleep quality involves practical steps. Set a consistent sleep schedule, aiming for the recommended duration. Create a sleep-friendly environment by keeping your bedroom cool, dark, and quiet. Practice relaxation techniques like deep breathing or progressive muscle relaxation before bedtime. Dietary choices, like avoiding heavy meals close to bedtime and limiting caffeine intake, can also influence sleep quality. Exercise itself can improve sleep when performed regularly, but avoid intense workouts close to bedtime, as they can be stimulating.

You should now have a decent understanding of how exercise and sleep impact Type 2 diabetes. Armed with facts and specific examples, you can make informed choices to leverage their influence for better diabetes management, fostering a healthier and more balanced life.

5

Weight Loss

This chapter explores the pivotal topic of weight loss and its direct impact on managing Type 2 diabetes. Let's explore the effects of excess weight when living with diabetes and provide practical strategies for achieving and sustaining weight loss.

Effects of being overweight with diabetes

Being overweight or obese significantly complicates the management of Type 2 diabetes. For instance, consider that for every pound of excess weight, your body's insulin resistance may increase. If you're carrying an extra 20 pounds, that's a substantial additional burden on your body's insulin production and utilization. This can translate to elevated blood sugar levels, escalating your diabetes management challenges.

Moreover, excess weight, especially when concentrated around the abdomen, heightens the risk of cardiovascular complications, like heart disease and hypertension. The interplay between excess weight and diabetes can also lead to kidney problems, nerve damage, and vision issues. The connection between these health issues and weight isn't mere speculation; it's well-documented in medical research.

Managing weight loss

The journey to effective weight loss is varied, and we'll explore practical strategies for lasting success. Consider setting realistic goals, like aiming to lose 1-2 pounds per week, which is both achievable and safe. Adopt a balanced diet that emphasizes whole foods, lean proteins, fruits, and vegetables. You can visualize this with examples like swapping a sugary breakfast cereal for oatmeal topped with fresh berries and nuts.

Portion control is very important; for instance, instead of devouring a large restaurant meal in one sitting, you can split it, saving half for later. Mindful eating practices, such as savoring each bite and recognizing hunger cues, can help you maintain a healthy relationship with food. Tracking your progress, whether through a journal or an app, provides objective insights into your eating habits and helps you stay on course.

Seek support from healthcare professionals, diabetes educators, or weight loss support groups. Enlisting the help of a registered dietitian can offer personalized guidance and meal plans tailored to your needs. Friends and family can also provide invaluable encouragement and accountability.

This chapter should give you an understanding of how excess weight can complicate Type 2 diabetes management, as well as practical strategies for starting and sustaining successful weight loss. With these facts and examples at your disposal, you can embark on a journey to shed excess pounds and ease the burdens of diabetes, potentially even reversing its effects.

6

Reducing Stress

This chapter focuses on the critical topic of stress and its significant impact on managing Type 2 diabetes. Let's explore the effects of stress, learn to recognize its triggers, and develop practical strategies to mitigate it, backed by facts and real-world solutions.

Recognizing Stress Triggers

Stress can have a profound impact on your Type 2 diabetes management. Consider this fact: when stressed, your body releases stress hormones like cortisol, which can cause blood sugar levels to spike. Identifying stress triggers is crucial for effective stress management. Some common stressors include:

- Work-related pressures affecting approximately 80% of people.
- Financial worries, which impact nearly 72% of adults.
- Daily hassles like traffic jams, leading to a 33% increase in stress levels.

Developing Strategies to Reduce Stress in Your Life

Reducing stress involves actionable steps. When faced with stressors, effective problem-solving techniques can be your lifeline. For instance, if work-related stress is your trigger, consider negotiating workload or setting boundaries to regain control. Some strategies to reduce stress include:

- Time management techniques like creating to-do lists and prioritizing tasks.
- Setting realistic expectations and learning to say no to lessen pressure.

Practical Types of Meditation

Meditation is a potent tool for stress reduction, and various types can suit your preferences and lifestyle. Consider these practical meditation types, each backed by research for stress management:

- **Mindfulness meditation**: Grounded in the present moment, it reduces stress by 38%, according to a study published in JAMA Internal Medicine.
- **Guided imagery**: Visualizing peaceful scenes or positive outcomes can reduce anxiety and stress by up to 25%, as reported by the American Psychological Association.
- **Progressive muscle relaxation**: This technique has been shown to lower stress and improve sleep quality (Harvard Medical School).

Exercise Ideas

Regular physical activity not only benefits your physical health but also has a direct impact on stress reduction. Here are some exercise ideas to consider:

- **Yoga**: Combines physical postures, breathing exercises, and meditation techniques.
- **Running**: Provides an invigorating way to reduce stress and improve mood.
- **Dancing**: An enjoyable way to get moving and relieve stress.
- **Weight Training**: An excellent way of reducing stress while lowering blood sugar levels.

Hobbies

Engaging in hobbies provides a therapeutic escape from stress. Consider exploring the following hobbies:

- **Painting or crafting**: Creative activities that can lower cortisol levels.
- **Gardening**: A relaxing and stress-reducing hobby with documented benefits.
- **Playing a musical instrument**: A way to express yourself and unwind.

By the end of this chapter, you'll not only understand the tangible effects of stress on Type 2 diabetes but also possess a toolkit of practical strategies, meditation types, exercise ideas, and hobbies. Armed with facts and real-world solutions, you can proactively manage stress to enhance your diabetes management and overall well-being.

7

Medicines and Supplementation

Metformin

Metformin stands as one of the most prescribed medications for Type 2 diabetes management, with a remarkable track record. According to the American Diabetes Association, approximately 120 million metformin prescriptions are dispensed in the United States annually. This medication is lauded for its efficacy in improving insulin sensitivity and reducing glucose production by the liver. However, it's crucial to be aware of potential side effects; approximately 30% of metformin users may experience mild gastrointestinal symptoms, such as nausea and diarrhea. These effects are usually temporary and can often be mitigated by taking metformin with food. Understanding how to manage these side effects is key to ensuring consistent medication adherence and, consequently, better blood sugar control.

Berberine

Berberine, a natural supplement gaining recognition for its potential in diabetes management, warrants attention. Some studies suggest that berberine can be as effective as metformin in certain cases, making it an intriguing option. However, it's imperative to consult with a healthcare professional before incorporating berberine into your diabetes regimen. This caution is due to potential interactions with other medications and the fact that berberine may not be suitable for everyone.

Chromium

Chromium, a mineral pivotal in insulin function and blood sugar regulation, offers promise. Research indicates that chromium supplements may enhance insulin sensitivity. Nevertheless, the evidence remains mixed, and the optimal dose and form of chromium require further investigation. It's vital to approach chromium supplementation cautiously, as excessive intake can lead to adverse effects.

Vitamin B1

Thiamine, or Vitamin B1, plays a crucial role in glucose energy conversion. Individuals with diabetes may experience reduced thiamine levels, making supplementation an option worth considering. However, it is essential to consult with your healthcare provider before commencing vitamin B1 supplementation, as excessive intake can lead to adverse effects.

Alpha Lipoic Acid

Alpha-lipoic acid, an antioxidant with potential benefits in reducing oxidative stress and improving insulin sensitivity, has garnered attention. ALA has been used to treat hardening of the arteries due to oxidative stress of Type 2 diabetes. Some studies suggest it may be particularly valuable in managing neuropathy symptoms. However, dosages and potential side effects vary significantly, necessitating professional guidance.

Gymnema

Gymnema, an herb with a rich history in traditional medicine for blood sugar control, offers potential benefits. Research indicates that it may reduce sugar absorption in the intestines and enhance insulin function. However, like other supplements, its use should be discussed with a healthcare provider to ensure safety and effectiveness.

Cinnamon

Cinnamon, a flavorful spice, has shown promise in improving insulin sensitivity. While it may not replace standard diabetes medications, incorporating cinnamon into your diet can be a flavorful and potentially beneficial addition. Healthcare providers often recommend discussing how to include cinnamon as part of a balanced diabetes management plan.

Banaba Extract

Derived from the leaves of the banaba tree, banaba extract has been studied for its potential to lower blood sugar levels. As with other supplements, it should be used cautiously and under medical supervision to ensure it aligns with individual needs and treatment plans.

In this chapter, we've taken a look at various medications and supplements essential to managing Type 2 diabetes. The statistical data and insights provided offer a comprehensive understanding of the prevalence and potential of these treatments. Always remember to consult with your healthcare provider before initiating any changes to your medication or supplementation regimen, ensuring they align with your specific needs and treatment plan for optimal diabetes management.

8

Better Blood Glucose Management

Testing Options

Effectively managing blood glucose levels is a critical aspect of Type 2 diabetes care. In this chapter, we'll explore various testing options backed by statistical data to help you achieve better blood sugar control and enhance your overall well-being.

Finger Prick Testing with Blood Glucose Meter

Finger prick testing, using a blood glucose meter, remains a widely adopted method for monitoring blood glucose levels. In the United States alone, it's estimated that over 13 million Americans with diabetes rely on these meters for regular monitoring, as reported by the National Diabetes Statistics Report. These portable devices provide real-time results, enabling individuals to check their blood sugar throughout the day. Frequent testing is associated with better glycemic control, as studies have shown that those who test their blood sugar regularly are more likely to achieve target HbA1c levels.

Continuous Glucose Monitors (CGM)

Continuous Glucose Monitoring (CGM) systems have been gaining significant traction in recent years. According to the Diabetes Care Journal, as of 2020, over 1.8 million individuals worldwide were using CGM's to manage their diabetes. These innovative devices offer real-time, continuous data on glucose levels, eliminating the need for frequent finger pricks. Studies have demonstrated that CGMs contribute to improved glycemic control by reducing both hypoglycemic and hyperglycemic events. The Diabetes Technology & Therapeutics Journal reported that CGM users experience reduced time spent in hypoglycemia and hyperglycemia compared to those using traditional finger prick testing.

Timing of Testing

Optimal timing for blood glucose testing is key to effective diabetes management. Consider these insights:

Fasting: Morning fasting tests help establish baseline glucose levels. Research published in the JAMA Network Open suggests that fasting glucose levels correlate with long-term diabetes outcomes.

Post-Meal: The American Diabetes Association recommends post-meal testing approximately 1-2 hours after eating.

Before and After Exercise: Monitoring before and after exercise can reveal the impact of physical activity on blood sugar.

Before Bed: Nighttime testing is vital, as nighttime hypoglycemia (low blood sugar) is a concern for many.

When You Feel Symptoms: Immediate testing when experiencing symptoms of hypo- or hyperglycemia is essential for prompt intervention.

By aligning your testing strategy with these insights, you can proactively manage your blood glucose levels, reduce the risk of complications, and enjoy a higher quality of life. The data-driven approach ensures that your diabetes care is both informed and effective.

9

Navigating Insurance with Type 2 Diabetes

Understanding how insurance works in the context of Type 2 diabetes is crucial for ensuring you receive the necessary care and support. In this chapter, we'll explore what is typically covered and what is not, drawing insights from insurance industry statistics.

What Things Are Typically Covered by Insurance?

- **Medications**: Most health insurance plans cover a range of diabetes medications, including oral medications and insulin. According to a report by the Health Care Cost Institute, in the United States, over 90% of individuals with commercial health insurance had coverage for diabetes medications in 2020.

  - **Medical Supplies**: Insurance plans often provide coverage for essential supplies like blood glucose meters, test strips, lancets, and insulin syringes. These supplies are considered vital for diabetes management and are typically included in coverage.
  - **Doctor Visits**: Regular visits to healthcare providers,

including primary care physicians and endocrinologists, are typically covered. The Affordable Care Act (ACA) in the United States has provisions that ensure coverage for preventive services, including diabetes screenings and counseling.

- **Hospitalization**: Inpatient care for diabetes-related complications or emergencies is generally covered by health insurance. Data from the National Diabetes Statistics Report indicates that hospitalization rates among adults with diabetes have been relatively stable, suggesting that insurance covers these services effectively.
- **Preventive Care**: Insurance often includes coverage for preventive measures, such as flu shots and vaccinations, which are essential for individuals with diabetes to prevent complications.

What Things Are Not Covered by Insurance?

- **Non-Medical Supplies**: While medical supplies like glucose meters and test strips are typically covered, non-medical items such as special footwear or diabetic socks may not be covered by insurance plans.
- **Alternative Therapies**: Some alternative or complementary therapies, such as acupuncture or herbal treatments, are often not covered by insurance. It's essential to check your plan's coverage for these services.
- **Certain Medications**: While many diabetes medications are covered, some newer or brand-name drugs may require a higher co payment or may not be covered at all, depending on your plan.

- **Experimental Treatments**: Insurance plans generally do not cover experimental or unproven treatments for diabetes. These are typically considered elective and fall outside the scope of standard coverage.
- **Weight Loss Programs**: Weight management programs, although important for diabetes management, are often not covered by insurance unless they are deemed medically necessary by a healthcare provider.

Understanding your insurance coverage is vital for managing the costs associated with Type 2 diabetes care. It's recommended to review your insurance policy carefully, including co payments, deductibles, and out-of-pocket limits, to make informed decisions about your healthcare. Additionally, staying up-to-date with any changes in healthcare legislation, such as the Affordable Care Act in the United States, can help you navigate insurance-related challenges effectively.

10

Untreated Consequences

T he consequences of untreated Type 2 diabetes are varied and can have a profound impact on one's health and quality of life. To truly understand the gravity of this issue, let's check out some specific statistics and the real-life implications:

- **Cardiovascular Disease**: Individuals with diabetes are at significantly higher risk of developing cardiovascular diseases such as heart attacks and strokes. According to the American Heart Association, adults with diabetes are two to four times more likely to die from heart disease than adults without diabetes. In fact, approximately 68% of people aged 65 or older with diabetes die from heart disease, and 16% die from stroke.
- **Kidney Complications**: Diabetes is a leading cause of kidney failure. The National Institute of Diabetes and Digestive and Kidney Diseases reports that about 44% of all new cases of kidney failure in the United States are attributed to diabetes. Moreover, people with diabetes are 10 to 20 times more likely to develop kidney disease than those without diabetes.
- **Blindness**: Diabetic retinopathy is a diabetes-related complication

that can lead to blindness if left untreated. The American Diabetes Association states that diabetes is the leading cause of new cases of blindness among adults aged 20 to 74 years. An estimated 28.5% of adults with diabetes aged 40 years or older have diabetic retinopathy.

- **Neuropathy**: Diabetes-related nerve damage, known as neuropathy, can lead to pain, numbness, and loss of sensation, primarily in the extremities. Statistics from the National Institute of Diabetes and Digestive and Kidney Diseases reveal that about 60-70% of people with diabetes have some form of neuropathy.
- **Amputations**: High blood sugar levels can damage blood vessels and nerves, leading to foot problems in people with diabetes. In severe cases, this may necessitate lower limb amputations. The World Health Organization (WHO) reports that every 30 seconds, a lower limb is amputated somewhere in the world due to diabetes.
- **Mental Health**: Diabetes can have a psychological impact. Expect to address potential stress, anxiety, or depression, and seek support when needed.

These statistics underscore the critical importance of managing Type 2 diabetes effectively. It's not just about controlling blood sugar levels; it's about preventing life-altering and potentially life-threatening complications. Knowledge is indeed power when it comes to diabetes, as understanding the risks of untreated diabetes can serve as a powerful motivator for people to take proactive steps towards better management and a healthier life.

11

Managing Expectations

What to Expect Dealing with Type 2 Diabetes

Managing Type 2 diabetes is a lifelong journey, and understanding what to expect is crucial for effective self-care. Here are some key expectations to keep in mind:

- **Lifestyle Adjustments**: Expect to make significant lifestyle changes. These may include modifying your diet, incorporating regular exercise, managing stress, and ensuring adequate sleep. Embrace these changes as essential components of your diabetes management plan.
- **Medications**: Depending on your specific needs, you may require medications or insulin therapy. Expect to work closely with your healthcare provider to find the right treatment plan tailored to your individual circumstances.
- **Blood Glucose Monitoring**: Regular monitoring of your blood glucose levels is fundamental. Expect to perform daily checks to understand how your body responds to different factors like food, exercise, and medications.

- **Fluctuations in Blood Sugar**: Diabetes is characterized by fluctuations in blood sugar levels. Expect occasional highs and lows, and be prepared to respond promptly with the guidance of your healthcare team.
- **Medical Check-Ups:** Regular check-ups with your healthcare provider are part of diabetes management. Expect routine screenings for complications such as eye, kidney, and nerve issues.

Managing expectations involves recognizing that diabetes is a manageable condition with the right knowledge and support. That's not to say it will be easy to make all the necessary changes required of us. It also offers an opportunity for a more health conscious way of living. By staying informed, adhering to your treatment plan, and seeking support, you can navigate the twists and turns of Type 2 diabetes with confidence.

12

Conclusion

I n our journey through "Living with Type 2 Diabetes," we've explored the various facets of this condition, from understanding its definition and causes to managing it with lifestyle changes, medications, and supplements. We've looked into the importance of blood glucose management, the significance of regular testing, and how to navigate the intricacies of insurance. As we conclude this book, let's summarize the key takeaways:

Living with Type 2 diabetes requires knowledge, empowerment, and proactive choices. By understanding the condition, its causes, and the importance of early detection, you're equipped to take control of your health effectively. Lifestyle changes, including diet, exercise, stress reduction, and weight management, play a pivotal role in diabetes management.

Medications and supplements offer valuable tools, but it's essential to use them under professional guidance. We've explored various options, from metformin to herbal supplements, each with its benefits and considerations.

Better blood glucose management is the cornerstone of effective diabetes care. We've examined testing options, from traditional finger prick tests to cutting-edge continuous glucose monitoring, along with the importance of timing in your monitoring routine.

Navigating insurance can be a complex but necessary part of managing your diabetes. Understanding what's typically covered and what's not helps you make informed decisions about your healthcare costs.

In closing, remember that you're not alone in this journey. Support from healthcare providers, family, and friends is invaluable. With knowledge, proactive choices, and a supportive network, you can effectively manage Type 2 diabetes, minimize complications, and lead a fulfilling and healthy life. Your journey continues, and you have the power to make it a successful one.

Thank you so much for reading *Living With Type 2 Diabetes*. If you found this book helpful and informative, I would really appreciate it if you left a favorable review for the book on Amazon.

13

References

Centers for Disease Control. (2023, April 18). *Type 2 Diabetes*. Centers for Disease Control and Prevention. Retrieved September 19, 2023, from https://www.cdc.gov/diabetes/basics/type2.html

How Type 2 diabetes progresses | ADA. (n.d.-b). https://diabetes.org/diabetes/type-2/how-type-2-diabetes-progresses

World Health Organization: WHO & World Health Organization: WHO. (2023). Diabetes. *www.who.int*. https://www.who.int/news-room/fact-sheets/detail/diabetes

Bidragsgivare till Wikimedia-projekten. (2023). Typ 2-diabetes. *sv.wikipedia.org*. https://sv.wikipedia.org/wiki/Typ_2-diabetes#:~:text=Diabetes%20mellitus%20typ%202%20eller%20ofta%20bara%20typ,samband%20med%20insulinresistens%20och%20relativ%20insulinbrist.%20%5B%202%5D

Fletcher, J. (2021, April 14). *Everything to know about carbs and diabetes*. Medical News Today. Retrieved September 19, 2023, from https://www.medicalnewstoday.com/articles/carbs-and-diabetes#foods-to-include

Felman, A. (2019, April 29). *How to count carbs with diabetes*.

Medical News today.com. https://www.medicalnewstoday.com/articles/317267#aims-of-carb-counting

Overweight & Obesity Statistics. (2023). *National Institute of Diabetes and Digestive and Kidney Diseases.* https://www.niddk.nih.gov/health-information/health-statistics/overweight-obesity#trends

Search results. (2023). Jama Network. Retrieved September 19, 2023, from https://jamanetwork.com/searchresults?q=Type+2+diabetes&SearchSourceType=3&f_SiteID=214&f_Categories=Diabetes+and+EndocrinologyANDDiabetes&exPrm_

Barnes, J. H., Eid, M. A., Creager, M. A., & Goodney, P. P. (2020). Epidemiology and risk of amputation in patients with diabetes mellitus and peripheral artery disease. *Arteriosclerosis, Thrombosis, and Vascular Biology, 40*(8), 1808–1817. https://doi.org/10.1161/atvbaha.120.314595

Yahoo is part of the Yahoo family of brands. (n.d.). Yahoo Search. Retrieved September 19, 2023, from https://us.search.yahoo.com/search?fr=yhs-invalid&p=guided+imagery+and+stress

Rd, J. K. M. (2023, July 12). *16 Simple Ways to Relieve Stress.* Healthline. Retrieved September 19, 2023, from https://www.healthline.com/nutrition/16-ways-relieve-stress-anxiety#4.-Practice-self-care

American Heart Association. (2023, August 22). *Diabetes risk factors.* www.heart.org. Retrieved September 19, 2023, from https://www.heart.org/en/health-topics/diabetes/understand-your-risk-for-diabetes

Eye complications | ADA. (n.d.). diabetes.org. Retrieved September 19, 2023, from https://diabetes.org/diabetes/complications/eye-complications